PAT DERICK

# COUNTING CALORIES

**The Essential Guide on How to Burn an Extra 500 Calories Every Day, Discover Effective Tips on How to Burn Extra Calories Without Extra Diet or Exercise**

**Descrierea CIP a Bibliotecii Naționale a României**
**PAT DERICK**
   **COUNTING CALORIES. The Essential Guide on How to Burn an Extra 500 Calories Every Day, Discover Effective Tips on How to Burn Extra Calories Without Extra Diet or Exercise** / Pat Derick – Bucharest: Editura My Ebook, 2021
   ISBN

PAT DERICK

# COUNTING CALORIES

**The Essential Guide on How to Burn an Extra 500 Calories Every Day, Discover Effective Tips on How to Burn Extra Calories Without Extra Diet or Exercise**

My Ebook Publishing House
Bucharest, 2021

# FOREWARD

There is an expression that I would like you to learn right now. This is an expression as well as a way of thinking that you must get in your head and it will help you in all areas of your weight loss journey. It will help you to reach your goal... whatever that may be.

Whether you want to lose a few pounds, or if you want to completely transform your body. The mentality I want you to program inside your circuitry is this:

---

### I'm Leaner and More Fit Today Than I was Yesterday

---

This simple, 10 Word Sentence is more powerful to you than anything else in this guide. This sentence should be printed and kept with you at all times. It should be your Mantra for the duration you spend on achieving your weight loss goals.

Failure to lose weight is as simple as being in the wrong mindset. The same could be said about completely transforming your body to that of the physical appearance you wish to achieve. You mindset plays a crucial role!!!

Believing the sentence above can, will and should become something you say at every meal, each time you wake in the morning, or before you shut your eyes to fall asleep... this is what will make your journey successful.

The times when you are about to fall off your "Weight Loss Wagon," this is the time you repeat your Mantra... and you will soon find that it becomes easy to stay the path.

And now that we have gotten the "Lose Weight With The Right Mentality" preaching out of the way... . Lets Rock!!!

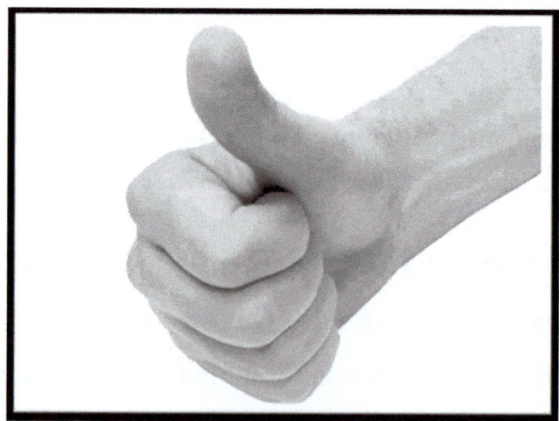

***I know why you're here.***

I've been there too.... and so have so many others. Millions and Millions in fact. That feeling of hopping from weight loss program and diet to the next. Following it to a "T" for the first few weeks and saying to yourself, *"I think I finally found a program I can stick with."*

Several weeks from that point your struggling again with eating unhealthy, or you have stopped losing weight, or you are craving a food that is off limits.

Next you fall off another program, and then soon the hunt begins for a new one, or you don't do anything and gain all the weight back that you originally lost. Just the thought of going back on another "Diet" makes you want to raid the fridge and eat whatever you can it is a vicious cycle.

They know it too... the weight loss and diet industry. The feed off of it to be honest… and there is no pun intended there.

Think about it; the weight loss and diet industry is a Multi BILLION Dollar a Year Market. Not a Multi Billion Dollar Industry... A Multi Billion Dollar a YEAR Industry!!!

In fact did you know that many of today's fitness and exercise magazines are actually owned by weight loss/fitness supplement companies.

It's no wonder people all over the world that want to lose weight and get into shape are so misinformed and have a hard time keeping up with and maintaining a good diet and or fitness regimen.

The weight loss industry wants to keep you confused and wanting more, they want you to think that what was great last month has been found inferior to the new information that was discovered most recently.

It's the information that keeps you from achieving your goals, staying confused and more important... shelling out your money to fill their pockets.

On the flipside I'm sure that you have a friend or family member, maybe even a coworker that eats like a slob, shoving anything that has a little bit of flavor and is edible and still maintains a great body.

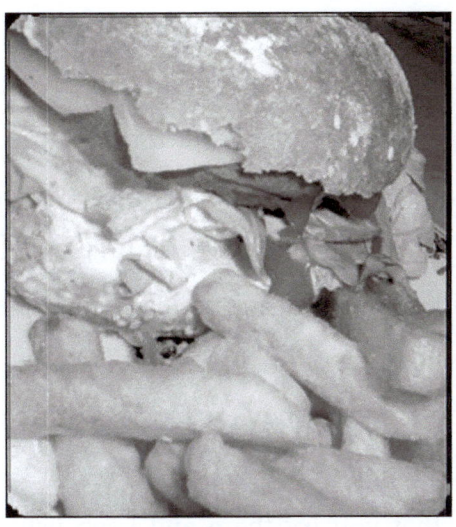

You may have even sat there with the person while they practically inhaled what appeared to be 15, 000 calories of fried foods, sugar, starch, cheese, and who knows what else.

In fact they may have even peeled the lettuce and tomatoes off their meal and commented "Eww, I hate vegetables."

You, sitting there with your salad, and small diet soda are left there smiling at them while you salivate over the juicy hot hamburger they are shoving into their mouth.

You watch in silent envy while they dip their fries in ketchup and devour the food you so wish you could have, but your current diet program says you cannot.

If this sounds at all familiar to you... rest assured you are not alone.

If you have been that person at the table or other side of the room watching this person with your top lip curled and gripping a fork in your hand like it was a weapon. I have some good news for you within the next several pages of this guide.

In this guide you are going to learn some very sneaky but successful ways to add some very small "tweaks" to your daily life that once you see what they are, and how effective they are... you will most likely doubt that they will work.

I only ask that you try them and keep using these secrets for several weeks and watch what will happen as you implement them.

One of the reasons you may have decided you wanted to read this guide was because you hate the idea of exercise and diet; however you know they are a necessary evil to get or stay in shape. Just the thought of running on a treadmill or picking up a weight makes you want to crawl in a closet and eat a box of donuts and think to yourself... "it's just easier this way," or "I just have to accept that I will always have a little more meat on my bones."

I have recently heard the term thrown around... "She's not fat, she's *fluffy.*"

As I said mentality is a lot in the weight loss game... you better come in prepared.

However if you're not quite ready to start working out on a regular basis and would just like to prepare by exploiting some "weakness in the fat loss armor, this guide will pave the way.

**'There Are Always Approaches to Make Things Work Better & More Efficient.**

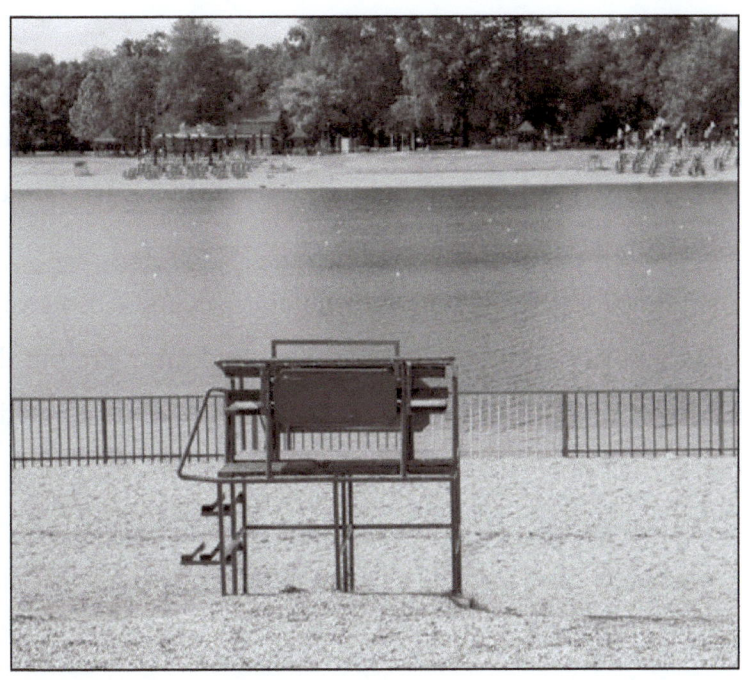

For example, if you were sitting on a beach and you wanted to get to the other side of the lake you could decide to swim to the other side.

This would get you there eventually and you could say.

"Yeah I just swam from that side to this side because I wanted to get here and see what it was like, but now I'm too tired to get back."

And now that you're on that side you realize that there is a boat with oars you can use to get back to your original side.

What are you going to do?

What is the more efficient tool?

Obviously the boat... but then again you could add a motor and then you really have the best way to get back to the other side.

Is it quicker yes... is it more efficient for you? Absolutely.

Can you say you took the long way to do it... no, but then again... how many times can you continue to work as hard as you can to get results that can happen 10x's faster.

That is the point of this guide... to show you how you can stop working so hard to achieve your weight loss goals, and start using some better and more efficient "tricks" to really rev up your calorie burning.

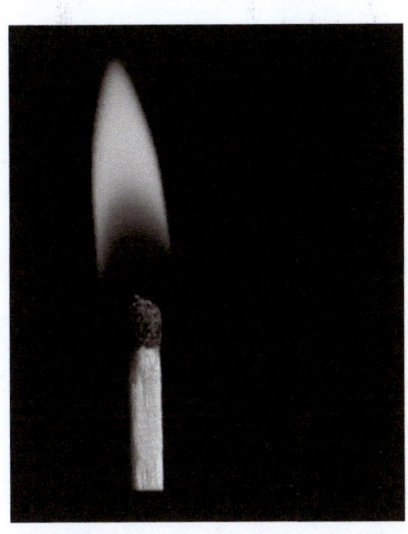

**So let's really get into it now... Ready!!!**

*So What Exactly is a Calorie???*

According to : *wordnetweb.princeton.edu/perl/webwn*

- a unit of heat equal to the amount of heat required to raise the temperature of one kilogram of water by one degree at one atmosphere pressure; used by nutritionists to characterize the energy-producing potential in food

Basically what that means is: How much energy it takes to heat up 1 gram or 1 milliliter of water by 1 degree Celsius

*Why is this important to you???* It gives you a better idea of what burning calories means. In its simplest form, when you eat food you are consuming something that is going to be required to go through a series of events as well as being used for energy.

The problem is when you consume too much and the amount of energy needed to be burned (calories) sit there and are continually added to... thus causing too many excess calories which leads to weight gain.

Hence to common weight loss dogma:

*To lose weight consume less calories, or burn more than you consume.*

In a nutshell: If you are burning more calories than you are eating, you should lose weight.

While this is fairly accurate... than why do some people eat WAAAAAAY more calories and still stay thin???

Some may say metabolism plays a part.

"She/He just has a better metabolism" or "She/He has a fast metabolism"

However there may be some other issues at work, and causes those people to eat junk food and still maintain a figure or body that people want.

It could be due to some things that a person does each day that you don't and it could be the reason why no matter what you do... it just doesn't seem to work.

If you haven't guessed already by all of this rambling. I will lay it out for you here.

Follow and Start to Use the Following Several Pages of "Tricks and Tweaks" on a Daily Basis... and You Will Start to Have Results.

**Tweak Number 1:**

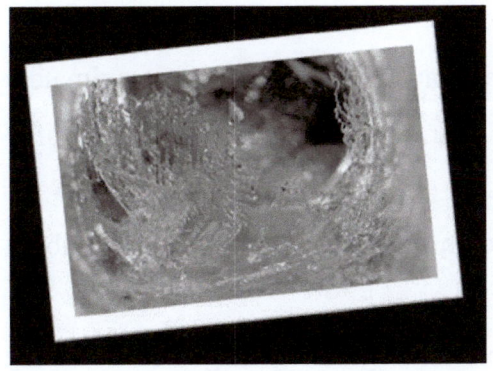

If You Drink Water...**Make it Ice Water.**

If You Don't Drink Water...**Start Drinking Ice Water!!!**

The average weight of an adult man is around 189 lbs (84 kg). We will call this man "Regular Average Joe" for the duration of this report because we will be mentioning him several more times throughout this guide.

I calculated that if an average man decided to start walking for exercise it would take him between 15-20 minutes to burn around 70 calories.

By using the Ice Water Trick and going by that common Drink 8, 8 oz cups of water a day... Guess What???

**You Can Burn The Same Amount of Calories Per Day!!!**

No extra exercise, no real big change in diet. Just Drink Ice Cold Water!!!

Just by doing this can cause you to burn approximately 25,000 extra calories per year, which equates to a loss of 7 Pounds (3.1 kg)

While this may not seem like a lot of weight, think about this.

If you use my example of Regular Average Joe weighing in at around 189 lbs (84 kg) in just over 2 years time if he gained around 7 lbs (3.1 kg) a year he would be over 200 lbs (91 kg)

Remember the definition of what a calorie is???

A calorie is how much energy it takes to heat of 1 ml of water to 1 degree Celsius. So if you drink 70 ml of ice water (64 oz) you burn 70 extra calories.

**Pretty Cool!!!**

---

**The great thing is…**

This is just One of the tweaks you can add…wait until you see the next one!!!

---

**Tweak #2**

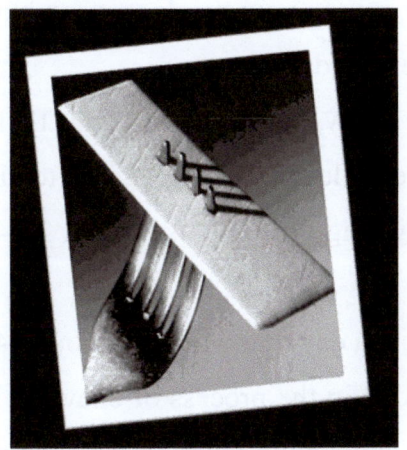

Start Chewing Sugar Free Gum After Meals.

This one is great because it attacks burning extra calories in 2 ways.

1. It saves you from consuming extra calories in between meals or planned healthy snacks.

2. You actually physically burn calories as you chew!!!

Yes I know it may not be a lot of calories burned by chewing, but anything is better than nothing.

The great thing is... I think you'll be pleasantly surprised at how many calories can be saved and burned if you chewed sugar free gum after meals.

Besides making your breath nice and minty fresh, or even better yet... sweet and spicy with Cinnamon gum; by chewing gum for several hours a day in between your meals you can burn and average of 175 extra calories per day!!!

See, for every hour you chew, you burn around 10-11 calories extra. Add that simple little chewing exercise to the calories you can save by not picking on foods is around 35-40 calories per hour.

If you chew gum for 4 hours a day you will burn around 40 calories from the energy expended in the process of chewing it, and around another 130-140 by preventing yourself from eating "pick on" foods or candy.

Add those together and you have saved yourself an extra 170-180 calories.

So let's go back to Regular Average Joe... let's see how much walking he would need to do for this amount of calories.

Regular Average Joe, just got home from work and his kids are yelling and screaming, he finds some bills on the table that need to be paid, and also finds out that his wife said the car needs to get an oil change over the weekend and there seems to be a noise coming from the washing machine.

Plain and simple... Regular Average Joe who just started this whole "I want to Stay In Shape" thing is now stressed, but he still needs to go out and walk to keep off another 170 calories.

He finds out that he now must find the time to get out there and walk an extra 40 minutes to keep those 170 calories from adding up.

Do you see how easy it is to have the effects of the day to day challenge you to just go out and do some simple exercises.

He now needs to find an extra 40 minutes to go out and walk... and he could have just simply chewed some sugar free gum from around 10 am-12 pm (lunch time) and then again from 3 pm-5 pm, all while sitting at his desk working.

Add in the ice cold water throughout his normal workday (1, 8 oz cup each hour) and he added another 70 calories to the day.

Sugar Free Gum + Ice Cold Water = 240 extra calories burned

But wait.... there's even More!

**Tweak #3:**

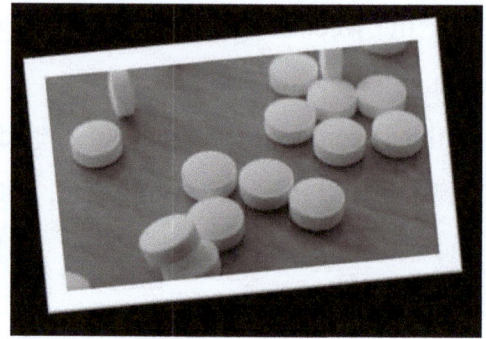

Add Some
Vitamin D to Your
Daily Routine

Due to Regular Average Joe and his hectic work schedule, it becomes very difficult for him to get out and see an adequate amount of sun during the day. The fact that much of his winter is also spent inside due to cold weather, it is no shock that Regular Average Joe may not get the required amount of Vitamin D in his body.

See sunlight can be used by our bodies through a process in which our skin more or less synthesizes the natural sunlight rays into useful Vitamin D for our bodies.

Did you ever notice the more sunlight you get, the more alive you feel... the more alert and awake you are. This is due partially to Vitamin D.

Not only does this awesome little Vitamin help to prevent some cancers, but research has also shown that it actually helps in a variety of other ways.

But in this guide... we want to know how it effects our calorie burning.

And Let Me Tell You... When you See How Much Vitamin D can help you may want to start calling it *Vitamin A+*

First you want to find a good Vitamin D supplement in pill form... this is the easiest and most efficient way to get the required amount of Vitamin D in your body.

The great thing is you are only required to take 1,000 IU per day. IU means "International Units" and is a standardized scientific measurement.

While this may sound like a lot... most Vitamin D pills contain this amount or more per little pill.

So if you want to take between 1000 - 5000 IU per day of Vitamin D, you can easily do this by taking just a few small pills per day, which will take you about 3 seconds to do.

So how many extra calories will taking this super beneficial vitamin burn throughout the day???

A Whopping 225!!!

Try Doing anything in 3 seconds and burn an extra 225 calories ©

So let's get out our calorie calculator for good old Regular Average Joe and do the math.

It's Saturday morning, it's raining and Joe wants to get his walk in before his normal day begins. He also remembers what his wife mentioned and remembers he has to bring the car in for an oil change, and the washing machine needs to be repaired.

He takes a deep breath while looking out his window and decides he is going to walk on the treadmill today instead of walking in the rain.

He sets his treadmill to his normal walking pace of about 2.5 mph (4.02 kph) and realizes he needs to walk for over 52 Minutes to burn 225 calories!!!

Almost an entire hour of being on the treadmill to burn the same amount of calories it takes to put a small vitamin in your mouth and swallow some ice water.

Speaking of Ice Water... he could actually wash down the Vitamin D pill with a nice 8 oz cup of ice water, and chew some sugar free gum afterwards, heck he can even do this while fixing the washing machine or waiting for the oil change to be done.

If he does this... he'll be at about 300 extra calories burned during that time, and has only added a these few tweaks.

Add them all together so far and if Regular Average Joe does all of the 3 tweaks on Saturday, he will have burned off a total of over ***460 calories!!!***

*460 calories burned per day,* by chewing some gum, drinking a small glass of ice water every hour or so, and taking a simple little vitamin.

If he decided to start doing these 3 tweaks on a daily basis for an entire year... he could prevent himself from gaining an extra 167,000 calories per year.

If you divide 167,000 calories by 3500 you get 47.7

Science states that there are 3500 calories in 1lb (.45 kg) of fat.

That 47.7 equates to 47.7 lbs (21.64 kg)

Are you starting to see how adding these small tweaks to your daily routine can keep you from gaining weight as the year goes on.

Now am I saying that if you do these 3 tweaks that you can lose that much weight each year???

Not exactly... but I can tell you that if you practice these 3 little tweaks you can prevent much of the weight gain you could if you did not introduce these tweaks to your daily routine.

And let's look at the people that I mentioned in the beginning of this guide that eat junk food all the time and still are able to maintain their body.

While they may not be using these exact tweaks, it is very possible that some of the things they do on a daily basis may account for many different reasons why they can eat that way and get away with it.

Let's also take a look at the normal "successful weight loss numbers."

If you have read about dieting before or fitness you most likely have heard that you should aim to lose no more than around 1-2 lbs (.45-.90 kg) per week.

Obviously this number can be more if you are very overweight; however the rule of thumb used in thousands of weight loss guides and diet programs are exactly that.

Now going back to my example of the amount of lbs per year (47 lbs) you may be wondering why I do not say that is generally what will happen.

It really depends on the person a perfect example is what the weight loss books say.

Think about it... 1-2 lbs per week would mean a person who diets would stand to lose anywhere from 52-104 lbs (23.6 – 47 kg) per year.

24

While there are some people that may need to lose that amount of weight, not everyone wants or needs to lose that much weight... so the numbers are relative to the person.

What I can say is that if you do practice these tweaks, they can prevent you from gaining weight much, much easier than by not implementing them at all.

Many times it is not so much about losing weight, as it is about gaining weight as time goes on.

Even with my first example with Regular Average Joe and just adding the Ice Cold Water. This could prevent a gain of 7 lbs per year.

If Regular Average Joe steadily gained an average of 7 lbs a year for 5 years, he would have went from 185 lbs to 220 lbs (99.8 kg) without really noticing.

It would be after those short 5 years that he would look at himself and say... . "What the Hell Happened to Me... I need to go on a Diet!!!"

The problem then goes back to: *Where do you find good information on a healthy diet, or even a fitness program?*

There are literally thousands and thousands of weight loss books on the shelves, some programs even have several books out just for a certain type of diet.

I wanted to share this guide with you so that you can make some small changes to your day to day activities that can help assist you in your weight loss journey.

I realize that weight loss for people is not a 1 size fits all method; however I can tell you that by following 1 or all 3 of these simple tweaks can really help supplement your efforts.

So now that you have learned some of these simple and effective tweaks let's talk a little about how you can pack even more punch to them for losing even more weight.

I do want to say that even though these tweaks show you how you can prevent weight gain, and possibly even lose a good deal of weight as time goes on without the need for exercise... exercise plays a very important role.

Many people make the analogy that exercise needs to be tough or it's not going to work.

On the flipside of that, there are many people that think that it is better to exercise at a nice leisurely pace for maximum benefit.

Regardless of which one is right, or which one is incorrect in your eyes, is not as important as picking some things you can start doing that you will **maintain** doing.

For regular average Joe I chose walking as the exercise he decided to do in my examples. Does that mean it's wrong if someone told you the better way to exercise is to jog, or do sprints instead of jogging.

The point is... Regular Average Joe chose something that he thought he would enjoy doing.

You may start to look at certain exercises and think to yourself "this looks fun, I could do this for a 1/2 hour or an hour."

The issue is however; once you start to do that exercise on a regular basis, you may find you dread doing it. Then exercise becomes more of a chore you *have* to do instead of want to do.

If you enjoy going outside and working in your garden, digging up vegetables or flowers, or raking it. If you move around and plant seeds in the garden and move throughout it weeding and making it look the way you want... is this a chore, or something you enjoy.

Did you know that if Regular Average Joe enjoyed gardening and did this for an hour or so every couple of days he would burn around 350 calories.

Are you going to tell me that gardening isn't good exercise if someone decided they hate to run so they chose to sit down and watch TV instead of exercising.

As I have said many times throughout this guide... Mindset plays a big role in the weight loss game.

Achieving and maintaining the correct mindset can and will only help you achieve your weight loss goals.

I want to give you a list of activities that many people would not think would be a good form of "exercise" and show you how they can help you achieve your weight loss goals faster than you may have previously thought.

These example will be based on Regular Average Joe, and a time duration of 1 hour per activity.

(Regular Average Joe = 189 lbs/84 kg)

| Activity | Calories Burned in 1 Hour |
|---|---|
| Acting | 257 |
| Body Surfing | 257 |
| Playing the Drums | 343 |
| Playing Ping Pong | 343 |
| Water Skiing | 514 |
| Dancing | 386 |
| Shooting a Basketball (playing OUT) | 386 |
| Playing Singles Tennis | 686 |
| Playing in a Basketball Game | 686 |
| Playing a Game of Kickball | 600 |

| Activity | Calories Burned in 1 Hour |
|---|---|
| Playing Catch (baseball, football, etc) | 214 |
| General Scuba Diving | 600 |
| Snorkeling | 429 |
| Roller Skating | 600 |
| Badminton Game | 386 |
| Canoeing for fun | 300 |
| Standing up and Playing Guitar | 257 |
| Surfing | 257 |
| Playing with Kids | 343 |
| General Skiing (snow) | 600 |
| Playing/Wrestling with Dog | 343 |
| Fishing | 257 |
| General Snowboarding | 446 |
| Hitting Golf Balls at the Driving Range | 257 |

Now these are just 25 things that I put together, and I'm sure that you could look at some of those things and find some really fun things to do.

I mean just think about when you go in the ocean and play in the waves... Regular Average Joe is going to burn over 250 calories, and he's having fun doing it.

If you want to take a look at where I have been gathering the activities and calories burned you can use this link http://www.caloriesperhour.com/index burn.php

It's actually really cool how it works, and as you can see very simple to use

## Activity Calculator

| Calculators | View List | View Results | Methods |
| --- | --- | --- | --- |

Weight: 189  lb ▼   Time: 1   hr  0    min

Search: [          ]   [ Search ]   mph ▼   in ▼

| Calculate | Undo | Clear | Kilojoules | Help |
| --- | --- | --- | --- | --- |

**Closing Thoughts:**

I hope you have found the information in this guide to be useful, but even more than that...

I hope you found the information contained on these pages to be a breath of fresh air. I hope that what you expected to read, and what you actually learned here did not only meet your expectations, but exceeded them.

There are many other ways that you can tweak and trick your body into burning more calories. Some require more work than others, and some require more time.

I wanted to create this for you as a "guide" or a supplement to whatever you decide to do to achieve your weight loss goals. I did not want to overburden you with a lot of information, and I tried to explain things so that not only would they be easy to understand, but also give you some knowledge that can help you move along.

We live in a world today where so much information and garbage is being thrown at us, that it's nice to take a moment to sit and just relax and learn something that is unbiased in a very biased and competitive industry.

Please take the ideas and thoughts in this guide and use them. I am familiar with many different tweaks and techniques; however the 3 contained in this guide are some of the most easiest to implement and can be started right now!!!

I wish you much success in anything and everything you do, and thank you so much for reading this guide.

Printed by Libri Plureos GmbH in Hamburg, Germany